PARENT ENGAGEMENT

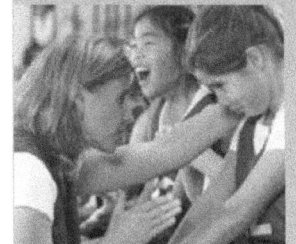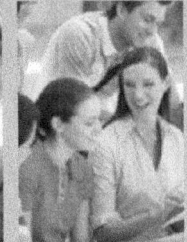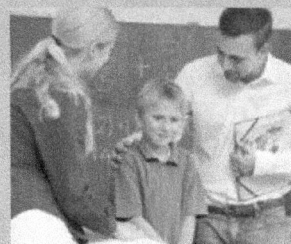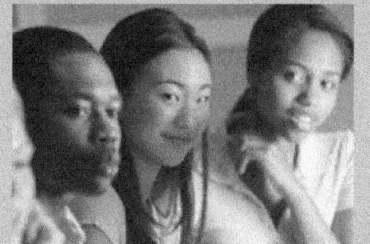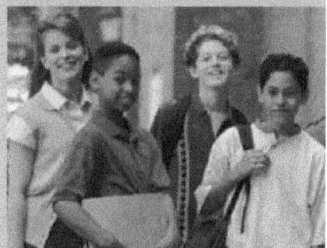

Strategies for Involving Parents in School Health

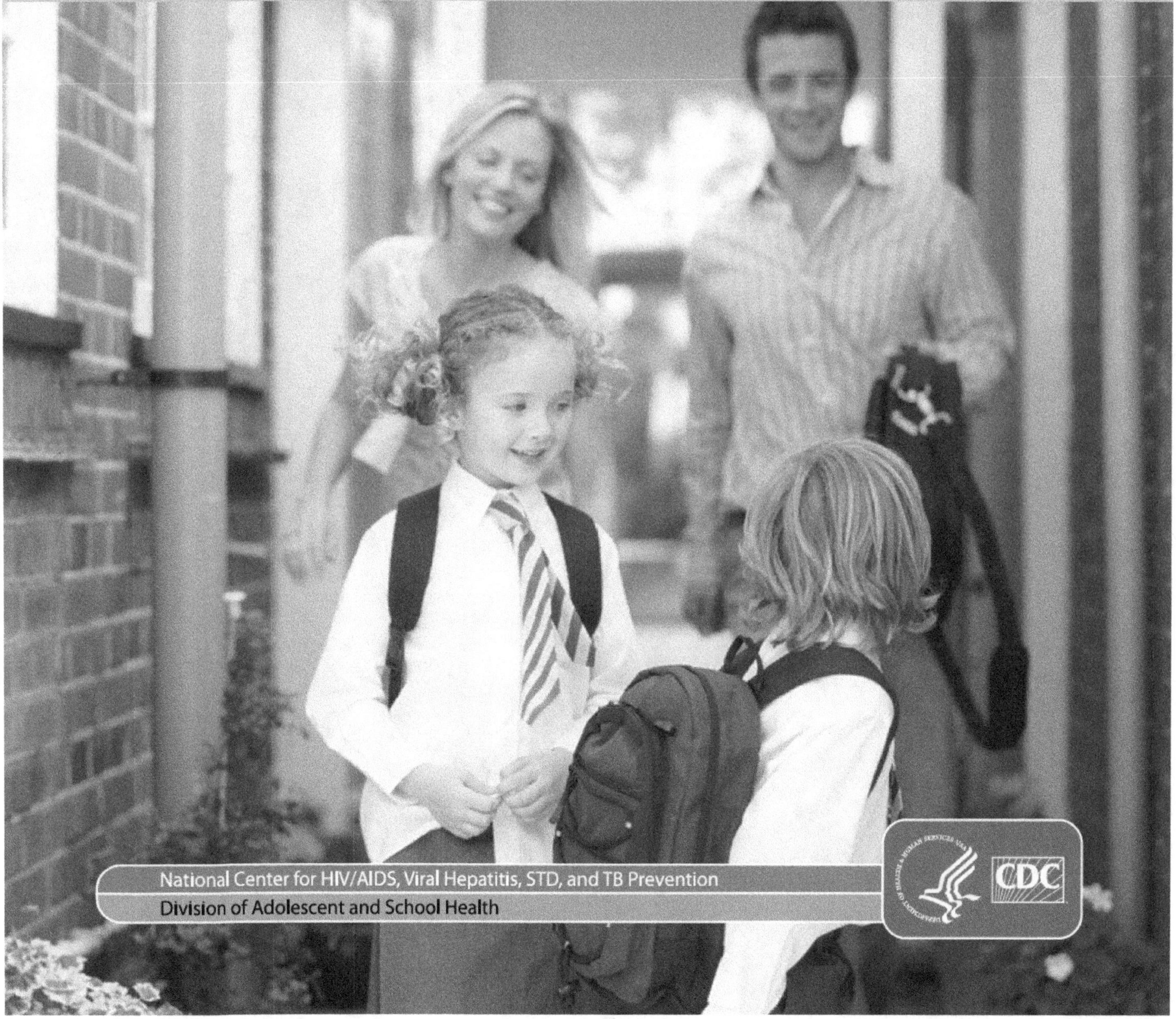

National Center for HIV/AIDS, Viral Hepatitis, STD, and TB Prevention

Division of Adolescent and School Health

 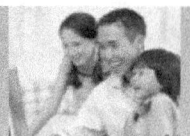

PARENT ENGAGEMENT:
Strategies for Involving Parents in School Health

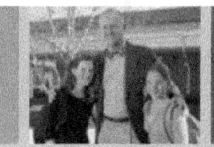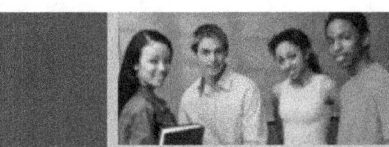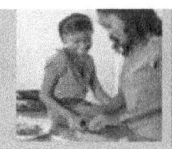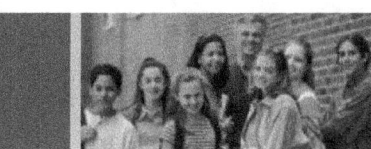

Suggested Citation:

Centers for Disease Control and Prevention. Parent Engagement: Strategies for Involving Parents in School Health. Atlanta, GA: U.S. Department of Health and Human Services; 2012.

To Obtain Copies:

Download from CDC's Web site: www.cdc.gov/HealthyYouth/

- Request by e-mail: cdcinfo@cdc.gov

- Call toll-free: 1-800-CDC-INFO or 1-888-232-6348

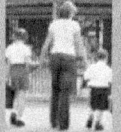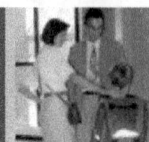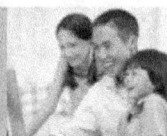

Acknowledgments

This document was prepared by the Centers for Disease Control and Prevention (CDC), National Center for Chronic Disease Prevention and Health Promotion (NCCDPHP), Division of Adolescent and School Health (DASH), with conceptual, technical, and editorial assistance from others across CDC and experts from the fields of health, education, and family involvement and engagement.

Parent Engagement Expert Working Group

Sarah J. Allen, PhD
U. S. Department of Education

Sharon Adams-Taylor, MA, MPH
American Association of School Administrators

Stephen Banspach, PhD
CDC, NCCDPHP, DASH

Lisa Barrios, DrPH
CDC, NCCDPHP, DASH

Sarah Butler RN, MSN, CDE, NCSN
National Association of School Nurses

Dana Carr, MPH
U. S. Department of Education

Chris Daniel
Families And Schools Together, Inc.

Twanna Davis
CDC, NCCDPHP, DASH

Patricia Dittus, PhD
CDC, National Center for HIV/AIDS, Viral Hepatitis, STD, and TB Prevention

Kate Eig
National School Boards Association

Joyce L. Epstein, PhD
Center on School, Family, and Community Partnerships,
Johns Hopkins University

Sue Ferguson
National Coalition for Parent Involvement in Education

Kari Gloppen, MPH
CDC, NCCDPHP, DASH

Brenda Z. Greene
National School Boards Association

Mary Haley
Action for Healthy Kids

Barbara S. Haywood, MSN, RN,C
Public Schools, York County, South Carolina

Pete Hunt, MPH, MEd
CDC, NCCDPHP, DASH

Sandra Leonard, RN, MS, FNP
CDC, NCCDPHP, DASH

Karen Lewis
National School Boards Association

Amanda K. Martinez, MPH, MSN, RN
National School Boards Association

Whitney Meagher
National PTA

Shannon Michael, MPH, PhD
CDC, NCCDPHP, DASH

Stephanie Neitzel
CDC, NCCDPHP, DASH

Ken Rolling
Community Learning Partnership

Linda Sheriff
National School Boards Association

Susan Shaffer
Mid-Atlantic Equity Consortium, Inc.

Sarah Titzer
Action for Healthy Kids

Liza Veto, MSW
U. S. Department of Education

Deena Zacharin
Office of Parent Relation,
San Francisco Unified School District

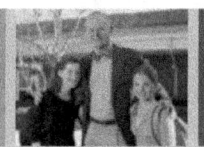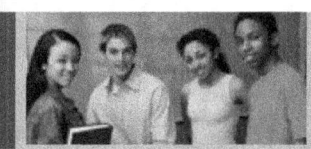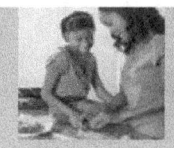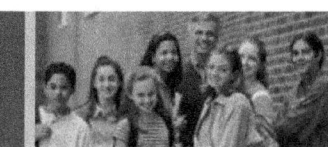

PARENT ENGAGEMENT:
Strategies for Involving Parents in School Health

Table of Contents

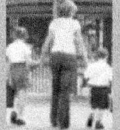
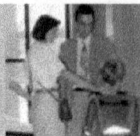
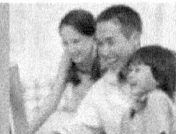

Introduction

Children and adolescents are establishing patterns of behavior that affect both their current and future health. Young people are at risk for engaging in tobacco, alcohol, or other drug use, participating in violence or gang activities, and initiating sex at an early age.[1] However, a growing body of research demonstrates that enhancing protective factors in the lives of children and adolescents can help them avoid behaviors that place them at risk for adverse health and educational outcomes.[2,3]

Protective factors include personal characteristics such as educational or career goals;[4] life conditions such as frequent parental presence in the home at key times (e.g., after school, at dinner time);[3] and behaviors such as involvement in pro-social activities (e.g., school or community sports).[5] Engaging parents in their children's and adolescents' school life is a promising protective factor. Research shows that parent engagement in schools is closely linked to better student behavior,[6–9] higher academic achievement,[10–12] and enhanced social skills.[2,9] Parent engagement also makes it more likely that children and adolescents will avoid unhealthy behaviors, such as tobacco, alcohol, and other drug use.[13–15]

This publication defines and describes parent engagement and identifies specific strategies and actions that schools can take to increase parent engagement in schools' health promotion activities. The audiences for this publication include school administrators, teachers, support staff, parents, and others interested in promoting parent engagement. Each of these audiences has different but important roles and responsibilities related to garnering support for, and implementing, these strategies and actions.

What is parent engagement in schools?

Parents play a significant role in supporting their children's health and learning, guiding their children successfully through school processes, and advocating for their children and for the effectiveness of schools. *Parent engagement in schools* is defined as parents and school staff working together to support and improve the learning, development, and health of children and adolescents.[16,17] Parent engagement in schools is a shared

responsibility in which schools and other community agencies and organizations are committed to reaching out to engage parents in meaningful ways, and parents are committed to actively supporting their children's and adolescents' learning and development.[16,17] This relationship between schools and parents cuts across and reinforces children's health and learning in the multiple settings—at home, in school, in out-of-school programs, and in the community.

For the purposes of this document, the word *parent* is used to refer to the adult primary caregiver(s) of a child's basic needs (e.g., feeding, safety). This includes biological parents; other biological relatives such as grandparents, aunts, uncles, or siblings; and nonbiological parents such as adoptive, foster, or stepparents. Parents guide the child's upbringing, which includes the interaction processes between parent and child that contribute to the child's emotional and social development.

How were these strategies developed?

The strategies and actions recommended in this publication are based on a synthesis of parent engagement and involvement research and guidance from the fields of education, health, psychology, and sociology. Materials in the review include peer-reviewed journal articles, books, reports from government agencies and nongovernmental organizations, and Web sites. Information from these sources was summarized to identify parent engagement practices in school that demonstrated an impact on students' academic and health behaviors. In addition, recommendations were informed by the opinions of expert researchers, public health practitioners, and educators at the Parents as Partners: Strengthening Parent/Family Involvement in School Health Policy and Practice meeting hosted by the National School Boards Association in 2008. This process identified evidence-based strategies and specific actions that can be taken to increase parent engagement in school health activities.

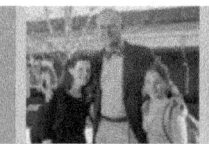
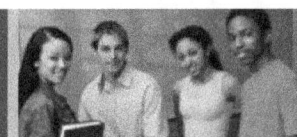
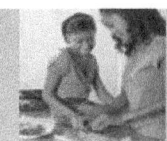
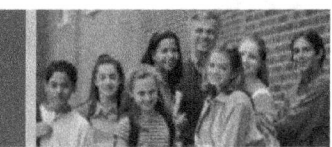

Only a limited number of studies have evaluated the impact of parent engagement on health outcomes. Therefore, many of the actions suggested in this publication are recommended on the basis of a single study of interventions that implemented multiple actions simultaneously, and it is difficult to isolate which components of the overall intervention contributed to observed positive changes in behavior and outcomes. However, actions were included only if experts from CDC and the panel of advisors for this project believed there was a logical connection between the action and parent engagement; the action was consistent with recognized standards of practice and feasible for most schools to implement; and the action was considered highly unlikely to be harmful to students.

Why is parent engagement in schools important?

Parent engagement in schools can promote positive health behaviors among children and adolescents. For example, students who feel supported by their parents are less likely to experience emotional distress, practice unhealthy eating behaviors, consider or attempt suicide, or disengage from school and learning.[3,18] In addition, school efforts to promote health among students have been shown to be more successful when parents are involved. For instance, studies have shown that when parents volunteer at their children's school, the likelihood of their children initiating smoking decreases,[14] and the likelihood of their children meeting the guidelines for physical activity increases.[19] In addition, interventions with a parent engagement component have been shown to increase positive health behaviors such as children's school-related physical activity.[20]

School efforts to promote parent engagement can be part of a *coordinated school health framework*. A coordinated school health framework engages families and is based on community needs, resources, and standards. In addition, this framework uses a comprehensive approach to school health by recognizing the importance of modeling healthy behaviors through staff health promotion and considering parent engagement to be an integral part of child

and adolescent health promotion at school.[21] When parents and schools work together, they can deliver clear, consistent messages to children, encourage the development of positive health and academic behaviors

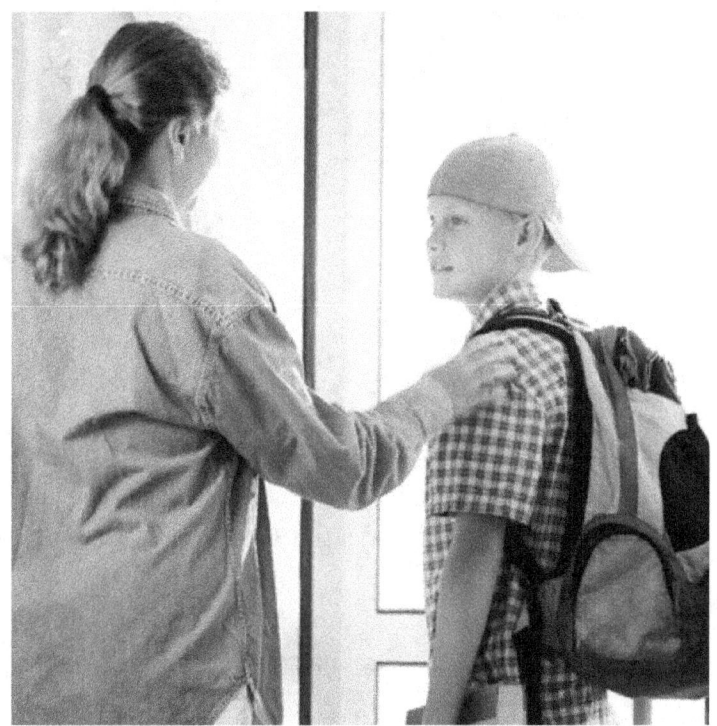

among children, encourage children to value education, assist children in getting necessary preventive care, and improve access to resources and support networks.[2,13,14,21]

How can school staff increase parent engagement in school health?

Although relatively little is known about what factors motivate parents to become engaged in their children's education, the primary motivation for parents to become involved appears to be a belief that their actions will improve their children's learning and well-being.[22] Therefore, school staff should demonstrate to parents how their children's health and education can be enhanced by their engagement in school health activities. In addition, parents tend to be more involved if they perceive that school staff and students both want and expect their involvement.[23]

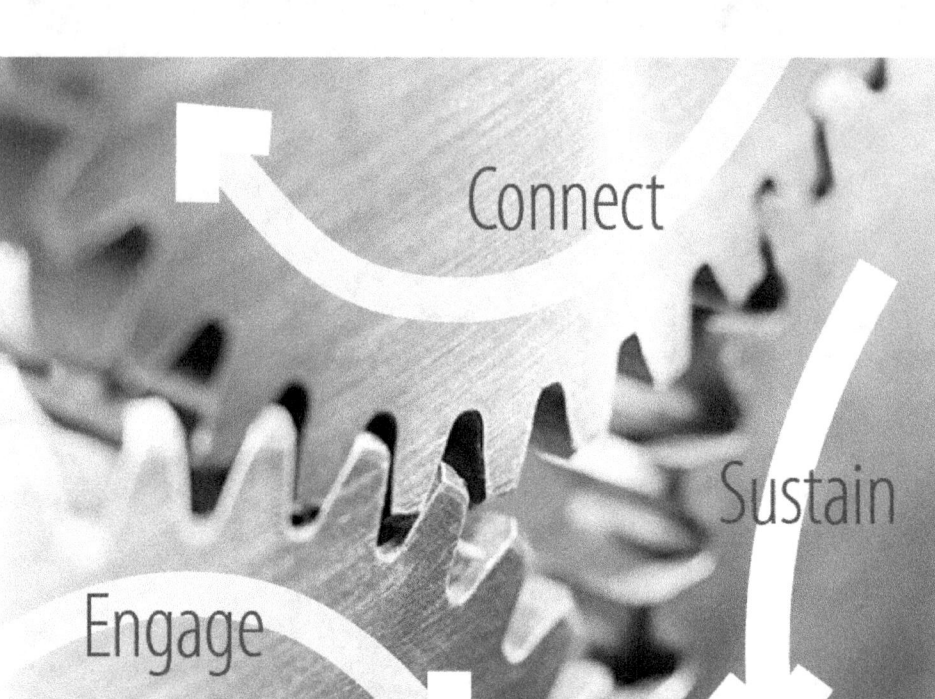

Figure 1. Parent engagement: Connect, engage, and sustain

To increase parent engagement in school health, schools must make a positive **connection** with parents. Schools should also provide a variety of activities and frequent opportunities to fully **engage** parents.[16, 24] Schools can **sustain** parent engagement by addressing the common challenges to getting and keeping parents engaged.

As illustrated in Figure 1, parent engagement is not a linear process, and the separation between strategies to connect with parents, engage them in school health activities, and sustain their engagement is not always distinct or discrete. For example, strategies used to connect with parents might overlap with those used to sustain their involvement, and schools might need to reconnect with parents throughout the school year.

Each school is unique, and it is not possible to develop one prescribed plan for parent engagement that is appropriate for all schools. The actions suggested in this document are not listed in order of priority and are not intended to be an exhaustive list. Some of the actions are small changes in school processes that can be done in the short term with relative ease, whereas others might be much broader, longer-term goals that require administrative or budgetary changes. Individual schools and school districts should determine which actions are most feasible and appropriate, based on the needs of the school and parents, school level (elementary, middle, or high school), and available resources. Schools should also evaluate their efforts to increase parent engagement in school health to learn which actions have the greatest impact.

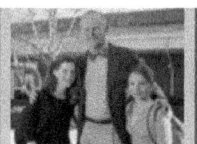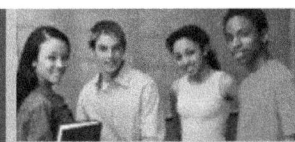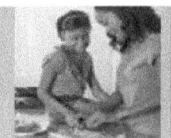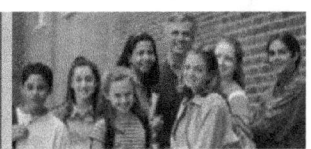

Additional Resources for Parent Engagement in School Health

Several organizations provide resources to improve parent involvement in schools that can be relevant to engaging parents in health-related activities. Schools can partner with organizations such as these to build on what is already available and reduce the burden of having to develop new resources for parent engagement in school health.

- Johns Hopkins' National Network of Partnership Schools
  www.partnershipschools.org

- Harvard Family Research Project
  www.hfrp.org/publications-resources

- Parental Information and Resource Centers
  www.nationalpirc.org

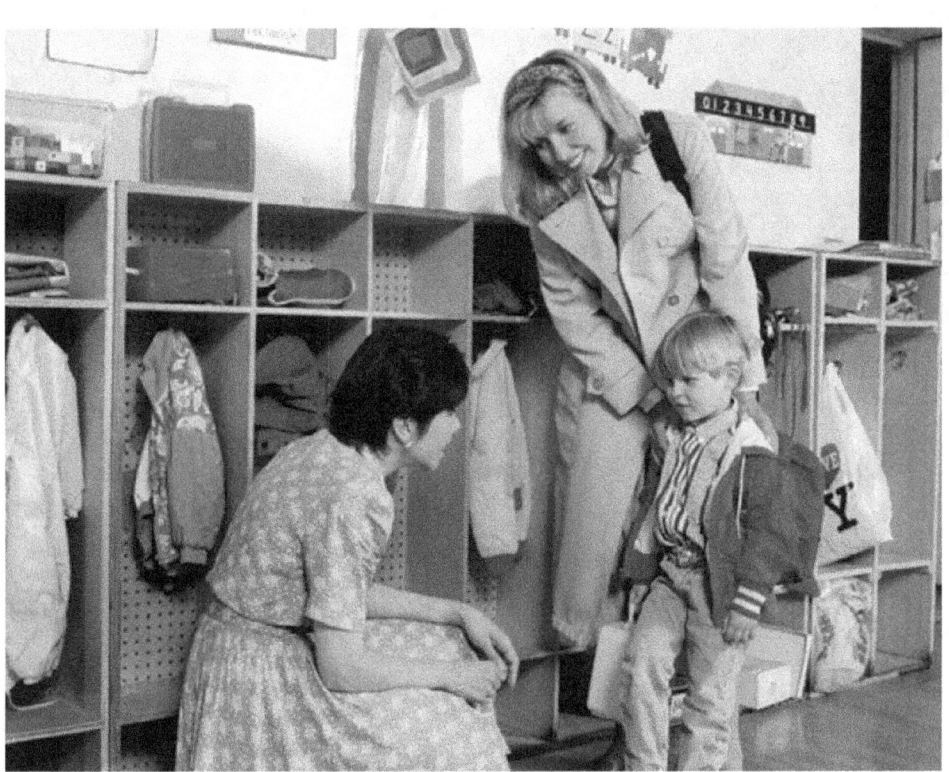

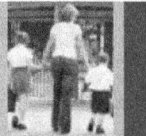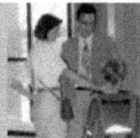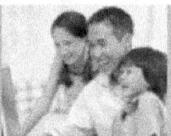

Connect

School districts and school staff need to *connect* and build positive relationships with parents before they can effectively engage parents in improving school health programs and activities. First, it is essential for school staff, parents, and community partners to recognize the advantages of working together to guide children's health and learning.[24,25] This can be accomplished by having a shared school vision for engaging parents in their children's education and communicating that vision to everyone in the school community. The school's vision for parent engagement can set the tone for a positive relationship with parents and the expectations parents have for being involved in school health and academic activities.

In addition, school administrators should assess the school's capacity to engage parents and establish or enhance policies and procedures for parent engagement. For example, school staff and parents can use CDC's *School Health Index: A Self-Assessment and Planning Guide* (SHI) (www.cdc.gov/HealthyYouth/SHI), a tool based on scientific evidence and best practices in school health, to identify strengths and weaknesses of school policies, programs, and practices related to family and community involvement in school health.[26,27] Results from using the SHI and the subsequent development of an action plan can help schools incorporate health promotion activities for engaging parents into their overall School Improvement Plan.

Furthermore, school staff should be prepared to work with parents. School administrators can enhance staff knowledge, ability, and confidence to engage parents by ensuring ample opportunities for professional development on effective parent engagement strategies.[28] For example, teachers can learn how to involve parents in students' health education homework or how to reach out to uninvolved parents. Schools might invite community partners to provide professional development in these areas and make staff aware of existing parent engagement resources. In addition, school staff can be given dedicated time to plan and organize parent-friendly activities and events.

Finally, school administrators and school staff should ensure that all parents feel welcomed in the school and should provide a variety of opportunities for them to be involved in school health activities.[29,30] School administrators might use a survey to assess the needs and interests of parents related to academics and health. The results from such an assessment can inform school administrators about the best ways to communicate with parents and help administrators prioritize the types of activities to implement throughout the school year to increase parental participation. An assessment also can inform school efforts to reach out to and engage parents whose children are at increased risk for chronic diseases and conditions, such as asthma. To ensure that all parents are represented in the assessment, school administrators should consider innovative ways to gather information from parents who are typically less engaged or who might not respond to school surveys.

Examples of ways school staff can connect with parents

Ensure the school or school district has a clear vision for parent engagement that includes engaging parents in school health activities.

- ✔ Does the school mission reflect the importance of parent engagement and establish a foundation for parent engagement in school health activities?
- ✔ Does the school have a well-planned program for parent engagement?
- ✔ Are policies and procedures in place to maximize parent engagement in the school's health activities, services, and programs?
- ✔ Does the school have a friendly, welcoming environment for parents?
- ✔ Does the school welcome parents to participate in and contribute to the school's health activities, services, and programs?
- ✔ Is there a district-level parent involvement and engagement plan that can guide the development of a school plan for involving parents in school health activities?

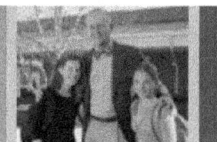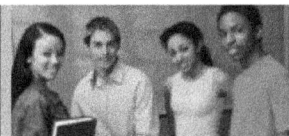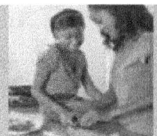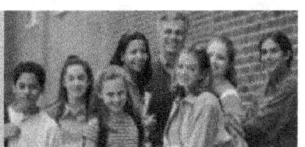

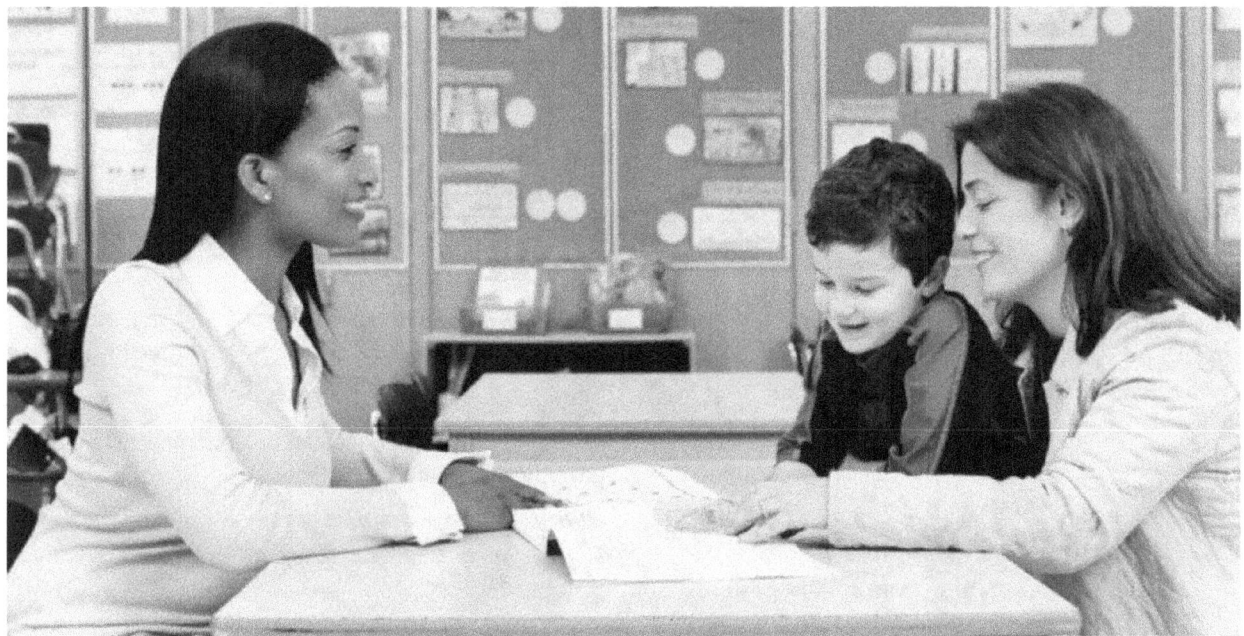

✔ Is there a district-level parent involvement and engagement plan that can guide the development of a school plan for involving parents in school health activities?

Ensure that school staff members have the ability to connect with parents and support parent engagement in school health activities.

✔ Does the school have a dedicated committee of teachers, administrators, and parents (such as an Action Team for Partnerships[24]) that helps the school plan, implement, evaluate, and continually improve its outreach to parents and the quality of parent engagement activities?

✔ Are there school health activities that address the interests of parents, such as healthy eating seminars?

✔ Are school staff members provided with opportunities to learn how to increase parent engagement in school, including in health activities?

Ask parents about their needs and interests regarding the health of their children and how they would like to be involved in the school's health activities, services, and programs. For example, the following questions might be integrated into an existing school assessment:

✔ What health topics are important to your family and your child?

✔ What information would you like to receive related to school health?

✔ What school health-related activities, services, and programs would you like to know more about?

✔ What simple changes or modifications would make the school's physical environment more pleasant, accessible, and safe for parents and community members?

✔ For parents with a child with an identified health risk, such as asthma, diabetes, or food allergies: how would you like to work with the school to most effectively manage your child's health condition?

✔ What skills and talents do you have that might match with the health-related needs of the school?

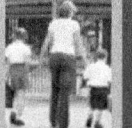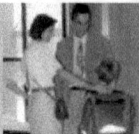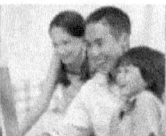

Engage

In addition to establishing a relationship with parents and making them feel welcomed, schools should offer a variety of opportunities to engage parents in school health activities. Researchers have identified six types of involvement that schools can use to engage parents[24]

1. Providing parenting support.

2. Communicating with parents.

3. Providing a variety of volunteer opportunities.

4. Supporting learning at home.

5. Encouraging parents to be part of decision making in schools.

6. Collaborating with the community.

The National Network of Partnership Schools (NNPS) has incorporated these six types of parent involvement into a framework for working with schools, districts, states, and other organizations.[24] This framework helps organize and sustain research-based programs of parent engagement needed to involve parents in improving student health and education outcomes.[16] Implementing activities that address all six types will increase the likelihood of engaging more parents in the health and education of their children in all grade levels.[16,31]

This section describes the six types of parent involvement as they relate to school health and gives examples for each. The examples are not prioritized and are not intended to be exhaustive. Rather, they are provided to encourage discussions within schools about how to meaningfully engage parents in school health activities. Individual school districts and schools should determine which actions are most appropriate for their school and community. Stories from the field are provided to illustrate how school districts and schools have effectively used these strategies and actions to engage parents in school health activities.

Provide parenting support.

School staff can build parents' leadership, decision-making, and parenting skills to support the development of positive health attitudes and behaviors among students and help build healthy home and school environments.[16,32] If school staff can enlist parents to lead and organize these educational opportunities, other parents are more likely to be receptive and willing to participate. In addition, schools that provide these opportunities and services to parents might get them engaged in other school health activities.

Examples of ways school staff can encourage healthy parenting support:

- Offer or collaborate with community organizations to provide parent education classes on the following topics:[8,14,33–36]

  - Understanding child and adolescent development.

  - Praising and rewarding desirable health behaviors.

  - Setting expectations for appropriate healthy behavior and academic performance.

  - Talking with children about health-related risks and behaviors.

  - Monitoring children's daily activities (e.g., knowing their children's whereabouts and friends).

  - Modeling healthy behaviors (e.g., taking medicine as directed, getting regular physical activity, and eating foods that align with dietary guidelines).

  - Strengthening leadership and advocacy skills.

- Provide parents with seminars, workshops, and information on health topics that relate directly to lessons taught in health education and physical education classes.[37,38] If the school has a school-based health center, encourage the staff to provide health workshops for teachers and parents. If the school does not have a health center, workshops might be

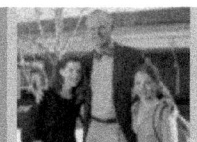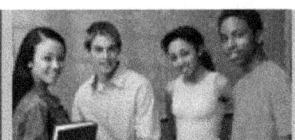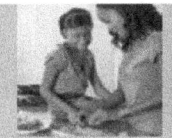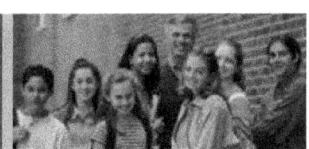

provided by other teachers; for example, some schools have a "health advocate," who is a teacher paid to ensure health-related curricula are taught. Schools also might be able to partner with community agencies such as local health departments to offer seminars for parents.

- Establish a parent resource center focused on child and adolescent health and other important family issues.[39,40] The resource center can be created and maintained through partnerships with organizations such as the health department, local hospitals, and other health and social service agencies.

- Hold school-sponsored, health-related activities in settings where parental presence is already high, such as in the neighborhood, at work, at community events, or at faith-based institutions.[36,41]

- Consider innovative options for reaching out to parents, such as partnering with local organizations to create a mobile parent center that provides education, health information, health screenings, and counseling services for parents.

- Offer school-sponsored health-related resources at local libraries and community centers and other venues where the families spend time.

Story from the Field:
Teaching Stress Management Skills to Parents and School Staff

In Buffalo, New York, at Early Childhood Center No. 61, the teachers and administrators believed that stress was holding parents back from becoming more involved in the school and that having more involved parents would benefit students. The school decided to offer a Sources of Family Stress and Relief workshop for parents and teachers. Parents of students in pre-K through fourth grade participated in the

event, along with teachers, administrators, staff, and community members. The workshop focused on stress management and coping strategies for parents to incorporate into their daily lives. Participants learned about exercising, relaxation techniques healthy eating, and sleeping. Dancing was also taught as a method to relieve stress.

Source: "Promising Partnership Practices 2007," National Network of Partnership Schools, Johns Hopkins University.

Communicate with parents.

Schools should establish clear communication channels between parents and school staff.[16,32] This can include opportunities for school staff to communicate with parents about school health-related activities (such as health education classes, screening programs, and other health-related events) and provide them opportunities to participate in school health activities and other community-based programs that focus on health. By

using two-way communications (school-to-home and home-to-school), parents can receive educational materials about different health topics, learn how they can be involved in school health activities, offer feedback and recommendations about health activities, and stay in constant communication with teachers, administrators, counselors, and other staff about their children's health.[16,32]

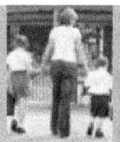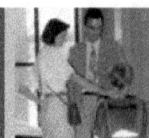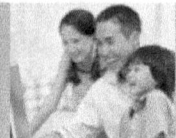

Examples of ways school staff can enhance communication with parents about health and education:

- Use a variety of communication methods, such as flyers, memos, banners, signs, door hangers, newsletters, report cards, progress reports, post cards, letters, monthly calendars of events, Web sites and Web boards, text messaging, and e-mail messages to communicate with parents about health-related topics and issues.[16,25,42,43]

- Use a variety of verbal and face-to-face communication methods, such as phone calls to home, automated phone system messages, parent-teacher conferences, meetings, school events, radio station announcements, local access television, television public service announcements (PSAs), conversations at school, and regular parent seminars to communicate with parents about health topics and issues.[16,25,42,43]

- Provide open lines of communication for receiving comments and suggestions from parents on health-related topics, and build the school's capacity to route this information to the intended persons. Establish multiple mechanisms for gathering opinions from parents, students, and teachers, such as on-site suggestion boxes, annual parent surveys, random-sample parent phone surveys, parent/teacher focus groups, and school-sponsored parent blogs.[24,44]

- Appoint or hire a school staff member (e.g., a parent liaison) to be the point of contact for parents in the schools.

- Communicate with parents about school health information and activities through non-school groups, such as faith-based and other community organizations.[24,44]

- Establish regular meetings with parents to discuss school health issues and children's behavior, grades, and accomplishments.[45–47]

- Create opportunities at school for parents to share important aspects of their culture, needs, and expectations related to the health of their children.[48,49]

- Create opportunities for parents of children with special health care needs (e.g., asthma, diabetes, or food allergies) to meet and discuss concerns and solutions.

- Translate health-related materials into different languages, or identify health materials already available in languages spoken by parents in the school community.[48] Provide bilingual interpreters to assist non-English-speaking families at school health events, and provide sign language interpreters for those who are deaf or hearing impaired.

- Provide information to parents when students are given health screenings in school (e.g., eye exams, hearing tests, or body mass index assessments) and suggestions for follow-up services.

- Ensure the school nurse works with parents to create individualized health care plans (IHPs) for children with special health and medication needs.[50]

Story from the Field:
Communicating with Parents About School Meals

To communicate school meal options, prices, and nutritional information with parents, the Shelby County School District in Tennessee implemented the Virtual Café, an educational tool for parents to use with their children. The Virtual Café is an online tool that allows parents to view the foods offered each day and help their children select healthy meals at school. The tool helps parents monitor the types of meals children choose and also includes a feature that allows parents and school nurses to select appropriate meals for children with special dietary needs. In addition, parents are able to prepay online for their children's meals.

Source: Alliance for a Healthier Generation, Success Stories Volume 23, April 2009 Newsletter.

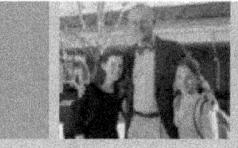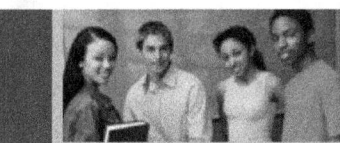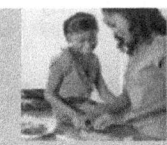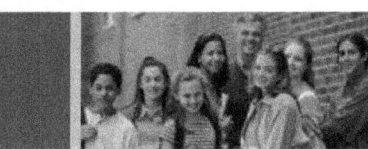

Provide a variety of volunteer opportunities.

Involving parent members as school volunteers can enrich health and physical education classes, improve the delivery of health services, and help create safe and healthy environments for students.[16,32] To maximize parent engagement, schools should offer a variety of ways for parents to become involved.

Examples of ways school staff can create opportunities for parents to volunteer:

- Encourage parents to serve as mentors, coaching assistants, monitors, chaperones, and tutors for school health activities.[21,23]

- Invite parent volunteers to lead lunch-time walks, weekend games, and after-school exercise programs in dance, cheerleading, karate, aerobics, yoga, and other activities that show their skills and talents.[51] For example, a parent who is a personal trainer might be willing to volunteer at a health fair, or a parent who is a gardener might be willing to start a school garden.

- Enlist parent volunteers to staff school facilities after school hours, allowing for community access to safe facilities for physical activity.[51]

- Involve parents in helping write health-related grants for the school.

- Enlist volunteers to coordinate phone call reminders to parents of their volunteer commitments, provide training, and organize volunteer activities and recognition events.

- Enlist parents of students with special health care needs (e.g., asthma, diabetes, or food allergies) to share expertise and experiences in staff meetings or professional development events.

Story from the Field: Increasing Volunteerism to Promote School Safety

As a way to increase student safety, John Humbird Elementary School in Cumberland, Maryland, instituted a program called Watch DOGS (Dads of Great Students), in which parent volunteers serve as in-school monitors and mentors. Forty-five fathers and father figures volunteered their time to monitor students in the school. Volunteers were given t-shirts to identify themselves as Watch DOGS and to increase visibility of the program. For several months out of the school year, there was a Watch DOGS volunteer in classrooms, on the playground, or in the cafeteria every day.

Source: National Network of Partnership Schools; Type 2; Fall, 2008, No. 25.

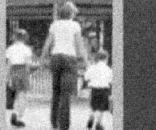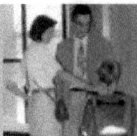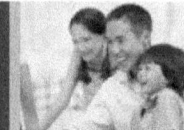

Support learning at home.

Schools can also engage parents and students in health education activities at home.[16,32] Engaging parents in homework assignments or other health activities at home can increase the likelihood that students receive consistent messages at home and in school.[52,53]

Examples of ways school staff can enhance learning at home:

- Train teachers to develop family-based education strategies that involve parents in discussions about health topics with their children (e.g., homework assignments that involve parent participation) and health promotion projects in the community.[28]

- Identify health promotion projects in the community that could involve parents. For example, invite family members to participate in physical activities at school or in the community, such as runs or walkathons.

- Encourage students to teach their parents about health and safety behaviors they learn in school (e.g., the importance of hand washing and of using seat belts and helmets).

- Ask parents to engage their children in health-related learning experiences, such as cooking dinner and packing lunch together, shopping for healthy foods, and reading labels on over-the-counter medicines.[54]

- Suggest ways parents can make family outings fun learning experiences and promote healthy behaviors (e.g., picking fruit or hiking).

- Host discussions about how parents can support healthy behaviors at home. Such discussions might be held at open houses and back-to-school nights, at parent meetings, and during parent-teacher conferences.

Story from the Field: Enhancing Learning at Home

Parma Park Elementary School in Parma Heights, Ohio, participated in PTA's Healthy Lifestyle Month by creating a bingo board contest. The bingo board included 25 squares of nutrition and fitness tips that focused on family friendly activities such as taking a nature walk, competing in a family relay race at the local track, avoiding fast food for a week, or making homemade applesauce together. Bingo boards were sent home at the end of October, giving students a month to complete an entire row of activities. Students who participated were then invited to a PTA-sponsored Fruit Smoothie Bar held at the school. In addition to receiving a fruit smoothie, the school held a raffle for prizes that included fun family activities such as a laser tag gift card, a family season pass for a local toboggan run, tickets to local a zoo, and a family activity coupon book. More than 150 students and their families completed their bingo cards.

Source: Parma Park PTA, Parma Heights, Ohio.

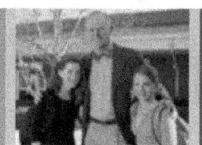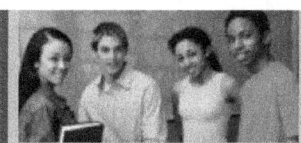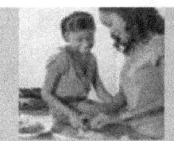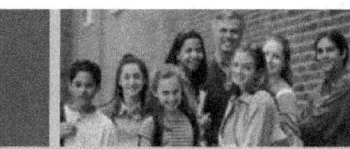

Encourage parents to be part of decision making at school.

Schools can include parents as participants in school decisions, school activities, and advocacy activities through the Parent Teacher Association (PTA) or Parent Teacher Organization (PTO), school health council, school action teams to plan special health-related events, and other school groups and organizations.[16,32] In addition, parents can serve on school committees or in leadership positions to assist with school decisions in developing school health policies, emergency/crisis/safety plans, health and safety messages, health curricula, food and beverage selections for school breakfasts and lunches, health services and referral procedures, and other plans and programs.

Examples of ways school staff can engage parents in decision making for schools:

- Involve students, parents, and community members in helping the school make decisions that improve the health and well-being of students through parent organizations (such as PTA/PTO),[24,44] school health councils,[21] school action teams,[24] and other school groups and organizations.[24,44]

- Involve parents in decisions when developing school health policies, emergency and safety plans, and health and safety messages; selecting health-related curricula or foods and beverages for school breakfasts and lunches; establishing health services and referral procedures; and other plans and programs.[51,55–56]

- Create policies that institutionalize parent representation on decision-making groups, such as school health councils.

- Provide parents with information about processes followed for health and safety policies: how they are developed, adopted, implemented, monitored, and revised, as well as the point of contact.

- Enlist parents in identifying school health and safety priorities (e.g., issues such as vandalism, violence, tobacco use, and drug and alcohol use).

- Involve parents in choosing health and physical education curricula with the help of tools such as the *Health Education Curriculum Analysis Tool* (HECAT) (www.cdc.gov/healthyyouth/hecat) and the *Physical Education Curriculum Analysis Tool* (PECAT) (www.cdc. gov/healthyyouth/pecat).[57,58]

- Give parents opportunities to be involved in developing or reviewing school health and safety policies, such as policies pertaining to alcohol, drug, and tobacco use prevention; injury and violence prevention; foods and beverages allowed at school parties; frequency of class celebrations involving unhealthy foods; and non-food rewards.

- Give parents opportunities to provide feedback on the meal program, and let them know the outcome.

- Give parents who have children with special health care needs (e.g., asthma, diabetes, or food allergies) opportunities to help develop or shape staff professional development events (e.g., educational sessions related to specific chronic health conditions such as asthma, diabetes, or food allergies).

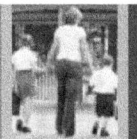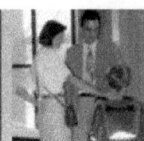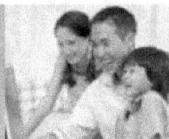

Collaborate with the community.

Schools can seek help with engaging parents in school health programs and activities from the community. In particular, schools can coordinate information, resources, and services from community-based organizations, businesses, cultural and civic organizations, social service agencies, faith-based organizations, health clinics, colleges and universities, and other community groups that can benefit students and families.[16,32] By working with community organizations, schools can help parents obtain useful information and resources from these organizations and give parents access to community programs, services, and resources. In addition, schools, parents, and students can contribute to the community through service.

Examples of ways school staff can collaborate with the community to promote parent engagement:

- Invite community partners who provide health services for students or parents to school or parent meetings to talk about their mission, services, and partners, as well as how they can collaborate with the school and students' families.[41,59]

- Create an agreement with community partners to develop and support school health programs and activities. This agreement should include how decisions will be made, how activities will be carried out, and how community and school partners will be held accountable.[41,59]

- Create a system that links families to community health and social service resources, activities, and events.[41,60]

- Collaborate with community partners to provide health services at school that meet the needs of students and their families (e.g., dental services, immunizations, health screenings, substance abuse treatment).[21]

- Link family members to school and community programs that promote health and safety, such as booster seat loaner programs, conflict resolution training, and mental health services.[61,62]

- Make school facilities available for use by community organizations that will host activities for students and their parents outside of school hours. The

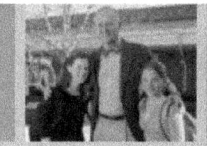 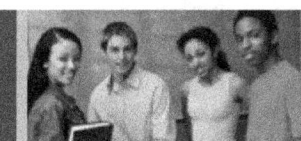 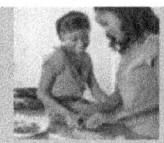 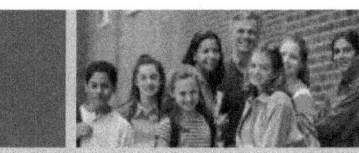

National Policy and Legal Analysis Network to Prevent Childhood Obesity (www.nplanonline.org) offers free resources on using school facilities for community use and developing joint agreements.

- Ask community partners to volunteer their businesses as vocational and community-based training sites or to host events at the school.

- Ask organizations or businesses to donate incentives for parent education programs and as gifts for parent volunteers.

- Encourage community businesses and organizations to sponsor service learning opportunities and other projects that enable students, staff, and parents to contribute to the health of the school and community.

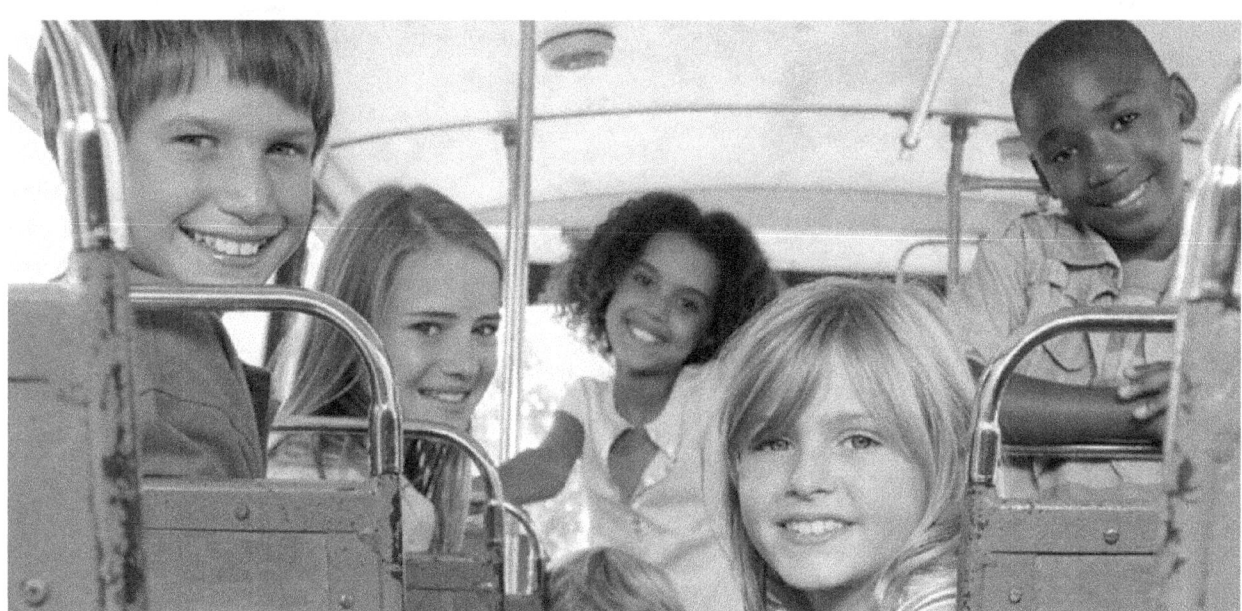

Story from the Field:
Collaborating with the Community to Ensure Asthma-Friendly Schools

The Albuquerque Public Schools (APS) Asthma Program in Albuquerque, New Mexico, works to make the city's schools more "asthma friendly." The program aims to increase student access to health care, ensure that every student has a designated primary care provider, help students obtain medications, and improve students' ability to manage their asthma effectively. This process requires collaboration among the school district, parents, and community organizations, so the APS Asthma Program created a community advisory board and linked with community health care providers. The program provided asthma education and management training to school nurses, mental health providers, school administrators and staff, and parents and community members at targeted schools and obtained feedback from trained recipients for continuous improvement. They also referred students and families unable to access state-funded or private health insurance to the New Mexico Department of Health's Children's Medical Services.

Source: Success Stories, Division of Adolescent and School Health, Centers for Disease Control and Prevention, 2007 and 2009.

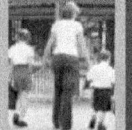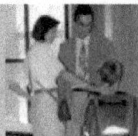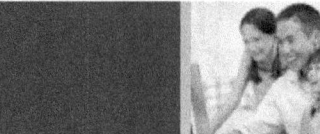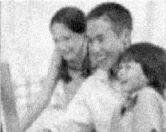

Sustain

If parents are engaged in school health initiatives from the beginning, they are more likely to stay engaged. However, keeping parents engaged can be difficult, especially as children grow into adolescence and move on to middle and high school. One important strategy is for school administrators and staff to identify challenges that keep parents from being connected and engaged in school health activities and then work with parents to tailor school events and activities to address those challenges. It is also important for schools to have a dedicated team or committee that oversees parent engagement.

This section describes six common challenges to getting and keeping parents engaged in health-related meetings and activities and suggestions for reducing or eliminating these challenges. The suggestions are based on expert opinion and field experience and are not intended to be in priority order or exhaustive. Each school's situation is unique, so some of the suggestions might work better in certain school districts or schools than others.

Solutions for six common challenges to sustaining parent engagement

1. Parents are unable to attend school health meetings or activities because of schedule conflicts (e.g., work, family, religious, and community activities).[29,63,64]

Suggestions to address the challenge:

✔ **Schedule meetings and activities to match varying parent schedules.**

- Survey parents to see which times/days are best for them.

- Schedule more than one meeting and activity opportunity.

- Schedule meetings and activities on a Saturday (offering teachers incentives for attendance).

- Host meetings and activities during the day for parents who work or are unable to attend at night.

- Host meetings and activities after rush hours.

- Host school meetings off school campus, such as in community centers or places of worship.

- Avoid scheduling meetings and activities that conflict with other school activities, major community events, and religious holidays.

- Offer a variety of opportunities and flexible times for parents to volunteer.

✔ **Provide incentives to encourage parents to attend at-school meetings and events.**

- Provide child care.

- Provide food or refreshments.

- Award door prizes provided by community sponsors. For example, schools can ask healthy food companies to provide gift cards to be used as raffle prizes.

- Make meetings fun with engaging activities and games.

✔ **Provide alternative ways for parents to access information and communicate with school staff, aside from attending meetings and activities on school grounds.**

- Establish an e-mail or listserv for teachers and parents.

- Create a phone number with 24-hour voicemail service for parents to voice concerns outside of regular school hours.

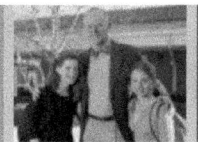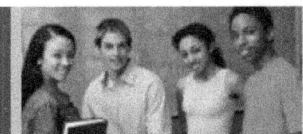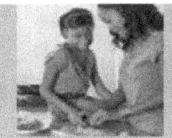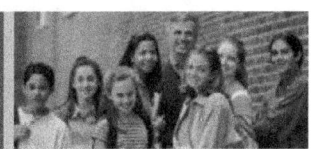

- Host a conference call meeting.

- Host a school blog or online bulletin board.

- Use forms of social media such as creating a secured Facebook page for the school, sharing updates via Twitter, and/or getting already involved parents to blog about school events.

2. Parents cannot attend school health meetings and activities due to lack of transportation.[43,64]

Suggestions to address the challenge:

✔ **Provide transportation.**

- Use school buses.

- Use a shuttle bus for different neighborhoods.

- For meetings that involve students and their families, extend school bus hours to pick up parents, too.

- Create a shared school community "ride board."

- Provide bus tokens or other public transportation fares.

- Arrange parent carpools.

✔ **Hold events off site or online.**

- Go places where families will already be such as community centers, community organizations, neighborhood centers or housing projects, libraries, and churches.

- Host online meetings with live feed (e.g., webinars).

- Create a podcast of a meeting and archive it online.

3. Parents are uncomfortable at school health meetings and activities. This discomfort might be the result of negative experiences when they were in school, unfamiliarity with the school culture, or other factors.[29,49,64–68]

Suggestions to address the challenge:

✔ **Provide opportunities for parents to get to know about the school and school staff in non-threatening ways.**

- Host events that provide information to parents on how the school works and how the school and parents can work together to promote the learning and health of their children.

- Host informal get-togethers.

- Provide continuing education opportunities for parents.

- Host parent-only social events at the school.

- Allow students to serve as greeters at school-sponsored parent meetings and activities.

- Have a designated greeter to ensure that every family is welcomed.

- Encourage teachers to schedule a first interaction with parents specifically with a positive, pro-student purpose.

- Invite parents to participate in a school meeting or activity at the school building before there is a problem related to their children.

- Promote the training and use of parent peer leaders and mentors.

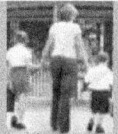 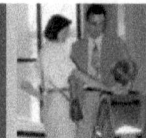 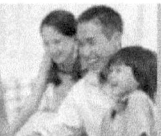

✔ **Implement programs that are culturally sensitive and that reflect the social and environmental aspects of a community influenced by race/ethnicity, socio-economic status, locale (rural, suburban, urban), and culture.**

- Assemble a representative group of all parents at meetings and activities.

- Host social and multicultural events to connect families.

- Promote diverse meals and healthy foods served at school meetings and activities.

- Ensure that multicultural and multilingual staff or parent liaisons are present at family meetings and activities.

- Host a broad community event that showcases all the different cultures in the school community.

- Set up international booths at school events.

- Encourage teachers to use textbooks and instructional materials that are culturally inclusive and relevant.

- Hire leadership and staff that reflect a multicultural school community.

- Make the school a de facto community center for families.

- Learn about and respect cultural values related to health issues.

4. Parents do not fully comprehend health information and communications provided at school health activities and meetings.[29,30,66] This might be due to language barriers (non-English-speaking family members) or unfamiliarity with terms used among those working in schools.[64,68]

Suggestions to address the challenge:

✔ **Provide translation services for non-English-speaking parents.**

- Provide translators at school meetings and activities (volunteer or paid).

- Ask parents or students (if appropriate) to volunteer as translators at school meetings and activities.

- Offer educational programs in families' home language.

- Provide school publications and Web site resources in multiple languages.

- Provide language-specific school telephone call lines for families.

- Host English as a Second Language (ESL) classes.

✔ **Reduce barriers to understanding information.**

- Avoid using professional jargon with families.

- Prepare materials and provide information at the 8th-grade reading level or lower.

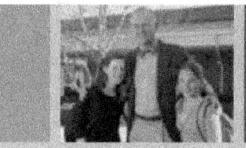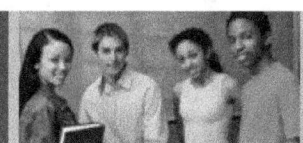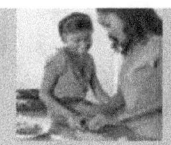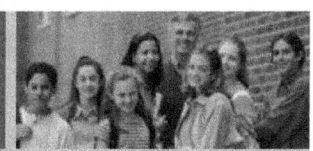

5. School staff are not experienced or trained to work with parents and have trouble sustaining relationships and parent engagement efforts. [63,69]

Suggestions to address the challenge:

✔ **Provide professional development opportunities for school staff that focus on strengthening parent engagement.**

- Offer a variety of topics (not all staff need the same professional development).

- Provide a flexible schedule for professional development to accommodate school staff members' schedules.

- Negotiate with universities to form partnerships and provide professional development, perhaps in exchange for doing research in the school.

✔ **Develop strategies for working through staff resistance to change, turf issues, and power struggles that might hinder teacher-parent interactions.**

- Provide teachers with sample/model assignments that include parents.

- Talk with school staff about their concerns related to parent engagement.

- Provide coaching to school staff on how to interact positively with parents.

6. There is difficulty sustaining school administrative or financial support for parent engagement.

Suggestions to address the challenge:

✔ **Share data with the principal that demonstrates parent interest and the positive impact parent engagement has on educational and health outcomes.**

- Share data on assessments of parent needs and interests.

- Present research that supports the positive impact of parent engagement.

- Present health data such as from the Youth Risk Behavior Survey (www.cdc.gov/yrbs) to show the health issues in the city or state.

✔ **Empower parents to speak up to school administrators about the positive impact of engaging parents in the health of students and the school.**

- Ask the PTA to communicate with the school administration about the benefits of parent engagement in school health activities and possible actions that can be taken.

- Invite school administrators, local media, celebrities, and school or health officials to attend school health events to witness parent engagement in action.

✔ **Seek opportunities for financial support.**

- Engage local college/graduate students to write grant proposals.

- Initiate strategies that require little or no financial support.

- Solicit funds from community partners.

- If the school is a Title 1 school, pursue funds from the 1% set-aside for parent engagement. Find more information at www.ed.gov/.

- Partner with a local PTA to apply for a Healthy Lifestyles Grant. Find more information at www.pta.org/pta_healthy_lifestyles_grant.asp.

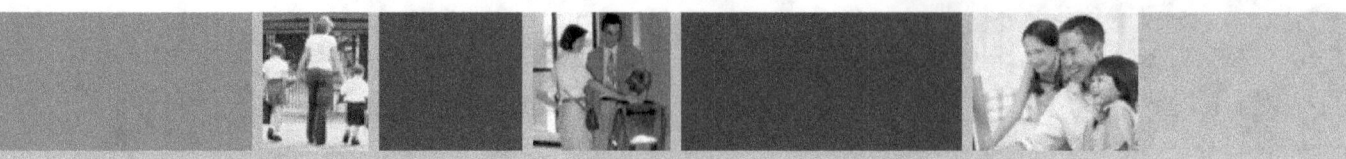

Conclusion

Research shows that students whose parents are involved in their education are more likely to have positive health and education outcomes than those whose parents are not involved.[2, 8, 10-12, 14] The strategies and actions presented in this publication provide a framework for how schools can connect with parents, engage parents in school health activities, and sustain parent engagement in school health activities. Parents, schools, and communities all need to work together to create an environment that facilitates the healthy development of children and adolescents.

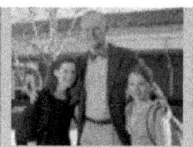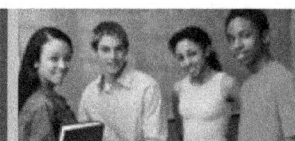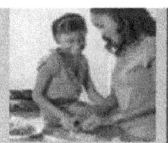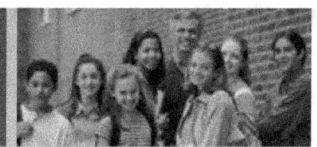

References

1. CDC. Youth risk behavior surveillance—United States, 2009. *MMWR* 2010;59(SS-5):1–148.

2. Hawkins JD, Catalano RF, Kosterman R, Abbott R, Hill KG. Preventing adolescent health-risk behaviors by strengthening protection during childhood. *Archives of Pediatrics & Adolescent Medicine* 1999;153:226–234.

3. Resnick MD, Bearman PS, Blum RW, Bauman KE, Harris KM, Jones J, et al. Protecting adolescents from harm. Findings from the National Longitudinal Study on Adolescent Health. *Journal of the American Medical Association* 1997;278(10):823–832.

4. Rosenbaum E, Kandel DB. Early onset of adolescent sexual behavior and drug involvement. *Journal of Marriage & the Family* 1990;52:783–798.

5. Blum RW, McNeely C, Rinehart PM. *Improving the Odds: The Untapped Power of Schools To Improve the Health of Teens.* Minneapolis, MN: Center for Adolescent Health and Development; 2002.

6. Epstein J, Sheldon S. Present and accounted for: improving student attendance through family and community involvement. *The Journal of Educational Research* 2002;95(5):308–318.

7. Sheldon SB. Parents' social networks and beliefs as predictors of parent involvement. *Elementary School Journal* 2002;102(4):301–316.

8. Flay BR, Allred CG. Long-term effects of the Positive Action Program. *American Journal of Health Behavior* 2003;27(1):S6–S21.

9. El Nokali NE, Bachman HJ, Votruba-Drzal E. Parent involvement and children's academic and social development in elementary school. *Child Development* 2010;81(3):988–1005.

10. Fan X, Chen M. Parental involvement and students' academic achievement: a meta-analysis. *Educational Psychology Review* 2001;13(1):1–22.

11. Jeynes WH. A meta-analysis: the effects on parental involvement on minority children's academic achievement. *Education and Urban Society* 2003;35:202–218.

12. Jeynes WH. The relationship between parental involvement and urban secondary school student academic achievement: a meta-analysis. *Urban Education* 2007;42:82–110.

13. Perry CL, Williams CL, Veblen-Mortenson S, Toomey TL, Komro K, Anstine PS, et al. Project Northland: outcomes of a communitywide alcohol use prevention program during early adolescence. *American Journal of Public Health* 1996;86(7):956–965.

14. Storr CL, Ialongo NS, Kellam SG, Anthony JC. A randomized controlled trial of two primary school intervention strategies to prevent early onset tobacco smoking. *Drug and Alcohol Dependence* 2002;66:51–60.

15. Guilamo-Ramos V, Jaccard J, Dittus P, Gonzalez B, Bouris A, Banspach S. The Linking Lives health education program: a randomized clinical trial of a parent-based tobacco use prevention program for African American and Latino Youths. *American Journal of Public Health* 2010;100(9):1641–1647.

16. Epstein JL. *School, Family, and Community Partnerships: Preparing Educators and Improving Schools Second Edition.* Boulder, CO: Westview Press; 2011.

17. National Family, School, and Community Engagement Working Group: Recommendations for Federal Policy. Cambridge, MA: Harvard Family Research Project; 2009. Available at www.ncpie.org/docs/FSCEWkgGroupPolicyRecs.pdf.

18. Resnick MD, Harris LJ, Blum RW. The impact of caring and connectedness on adolescent health and well-being. *Journal of Paediatrics & Child Health* 1993;29(Suppl 1):S3–9.

19. Ornelas IJ, Perreira KM, Ayala GX. Parental influences on adolescent physical activity: a longitudinal study. *International Journal of Behavioral Nutrition and Physical Activity* 2007;4(3):1–10.

20. Haerens L, De Bourdeaudhuij I, Maes L. School-based randomized controlled trial of a physical activity intervention among adolescents. *Journal of Adolescent Health* 2007;40(3):258–265.

21. Carlyon P, Carlyon W, McCarthy AR. Family and community involvement in school health. In: Marx E, Wooley SF, Northrop D, editors. *Health is Academic: A Guide to Coordinated School Health Programs.* New York, NY: Teachers College Press; 1998.

22. Hoover-Dempsey KV, Bassler OC, Brissie JS. Explorations in parent-school relations. *Journal of Educational Research* 1992;85:287–294.

23. Green CL, Walker JMT, Hoover-Dempsey KV, Sandler HM. Parents' motivations for involvement in children's education: an empirical test of a theoretical model of parental involvement. *Journal of Educational Psychology* 2007;99(3):532–544.

24. Epstein JL. *School, Family, and Community Partnerships: Your Handbook for Action.* 3rd edition. Thousand Oaks, CA: Corwin Press; 2009.

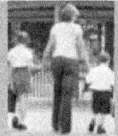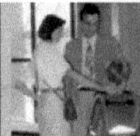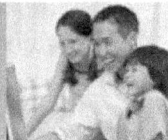

25. Henderson AL, Mapp KT. *A New Wave of Evidence: The Impact of School, Family, and Community Connections on Student Achievement.* Austin, TX: Southwest Educational Development Laboratory; 2002.

26. CDC. *School Health Index: A Self-Assessment and Planning Guide, Elementary School Version.* Atlanta, GA: U.S. Department of Health and Human Services; 2005.

27. CDC. *School Health Index: A Self-Assessment and Planning Guide, Middle/high School Version.* Atlanta, GA: U.S. Department of Health and Human Services; 2005.

28. Weiss HB, Kreider H, Lopez ME, Chatman CM, editors. *Preparing Educators to Involve Families.* Thousand Oaks, CA: Sage Publications, Inc.; 2005.

29. Gonzalez-DeHass AR, Willems PP. Examining the underutilization of parent involvement in the schools. *School Community Journal* 2003;13(1):85–99.

30. Winnail SD, Geiger BF, Nagy S. Why don't parents participate in school health education? *American Journal of Health Education* 2002;33(1):10–14.

31. Simon BS. Family involvement in high school: predictors and effects. *NASSP Bulletin* 2001;85(627):8–19.

32. Michael S, Dittus P, Epstein J. Family and community involvement in schools: results from the School Health Policies and Programs Study 2006. *Journal of School Health* 2007;77:567–579.

33. Haggerty KP, Fleming CB, Lonczak HS, Oxford ML, Harachi TW, Catalano RF. Predictors of participation in parenting workshops. *Journal of Primary Prevention* 2002;22(4):375–387.

34. Rollin SA, Rubin R, Marcil R, Ferullo U, Buncher R. Project KICK: A school-based drug education health promotion research project. *Counselling Psychology Quarterly* 1995;8(4):345–359.

35. Stormshak EA, Connell A, Dishion TJ. An adaptive approach to family-centered intervention in schools: linking intervention engagement to academic outcomes in middle and high school. *Prevention Science* 2009;10:221–235.

36. Miller KS, Maxwell KD, Fasula AM, Parker JT, Zackary S, Wykoff SC. Pre-risk HIV prevention paradigm shift: the feasibility and acceptability of the Parents Matter program in HIV risk communities. *Public Health Reports* 2010;125(Suppl 1):38–46.

37. Rollin SA, Rubin R, Marcil R, Ferullo U, Buncher R. Project KICK: a school-based drug education health promotion research project. *Counseling Psychology Quarterly* 1995;8:345–359.

38. Johnston R, Cross D, Costa C, Giles-Corti B, Cordin T, Milne E, et al. Sun safety education intervention for school and home. *Health Education Research* 2003;103(6):342–351.

39. Dryfoos JG. *Evaluations of community schools: findings to date.* Washington, DC: Coalition for Community Schools; 2000.

40. Knoffe HM, Batsche GM. Project Achieve: analyzing a school reform process for at-risk and underachieving students. *School Psychology Review* 1995;24:579–603.

41. Coalition for Community Schools. *Community and Family Engagement: Principals Share What Works.* Washington, DC: Coalition for Community Schools; 2006.

42. Chen H-m, Yu C, Chang C-s. E-Homebook System: A Web-Based Interactive Education Interface. *Computers & Education* 2005;49(2):160–175.

43. Hahn EJ, Simpson MR, Kidd P. Cues to parent involvement in drug prevention and school activities. *Journal of School Health* 1996;66(5):165–170.

44. Henderson AL, Mapp KT, Johnson VR, Davies D. *Beyond the Bake Sale: The Essential Guide to Family-School Partnerships.* New York, NY: The New Press; 2007.

45. Conduct Problems Prevention Research Group. The effects of the Fast Track program on serious problem outcomes at the end of elementary school. *Journal of Clinical Child and Adolescent Psychology* 2004;33(4):650–661.

46. Izzo CV, Weissberg RP, Kasprow WJ, Fendrich M. A longitudinal assessment of teacher perceptions of parent involvement in children's education and school performance. *American Journal of Community Psychology* 1999;27(6):817–839.

47. Quint J, Bloom HS, Black AR, Stephens L, Akey TM. *The challenge of scaling up educational reform. Findings and lessons from First Things First.* New York, NY: Manpower Demonstration Research Corporation; 2005.

48. Peña DC. Parent involvement: influencing factors and implications. *Journal of Educational Research* 2000;94(1):42–54.

49. Ryan CS, Casas JF, Kelly-Vance L, Ryalls BO, Nero C. Parent involvement and views of school success: the role of parents' Latino and White American cultural orientations. *Psychology in the Schools* 2010;47(4):391–405.

50. CDC. *Strategies for Addressing Asthma Within a Coordinated School Health Program, With Updated Resources.* Atlanta, GA: U.S. Department of Health and Human Services; 2006.

51. CDC. School health guidelines to promote healthy eating and physical activity among young people. *MMWR* 2011;60(RR-5):1–78.

52. Hoover-Dempsey KV, Battiato AC, Walker JMT, Reed RP, DeJong JM, Jones KP. Parental involvement in homework. *Educational Psychologist* 2001;36(3):195–209.

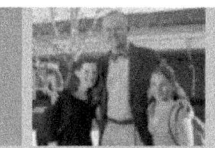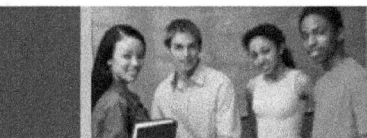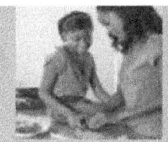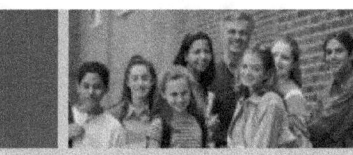

53. Van Voorhis FL. Interactive homework in middle school: effects on family involvement and students' science achievement. *Journal of Educational Research* 2003;96(9):323–339.

54. Blom-Hoffman J, Wilcox KR, Dunn L, Leff SS, Power PJ. Family involvement in school-based health promotion: bringing nutrition home. *School Psychology Review* 2008;37(4):567–577.

55. CDC. School health guidelines for school health programs to prevent tobacco use and addiction. *MMWR* 1994;43(RR-2):1–18.

56. CDC. School health guidelines to prevent unintentional injuries and violence. *MMWR* 2001;50(RR-22):1–73.

57. CDC. *Physical Education Curriculum Analysis Tool.* Atlanta, GA: U.S. Department of Health and Human Services; 2006.

58. CDC. *Health Education Curriculum Analysis Tool.* Atlanta, GA: U.S. Department of Health and Human Services; 2007.

59. Hands C. *It's who you know and what you know: the process of creating partnerships between schools and communities.* School Community Journal 2005;15(2):63–84.

60. Gold E, Simon E, Brown C. *Successful Community Organizing for School Reform.* Chicago, IL: Cross City Campaign for Urban School Reform; 2002.

61. McDonald L, Sayger TV. Impact of a family and school based prevention program on protective factors for high risk youth. *Drugs & Society* 1998;12(1-2):61–85.

62. Tremblay RE, Pagani-Kurtz L, Masse LC, Vitaro F, Pihl RO. A bimodal preventive intervention for disruptive kindergarten boys: its impact through mid-adolescence. *Journal of Consulting and Clinical Psychology* 1995;63:560–568.

63. Birch DA, Hallock BA. Parent involvement in seventh grade school health education: a statewide view. *Journal of Health Education* 1999;30(2):110–114.

64. Garcia-Dominic O, Wray LA, Treviño RP, Hernandez AE, Yin Z, Ulbrecht JS. Identifying barriers that hinder onsite parental involvement in a school-based health promotion program. *Health Promotion Practice* 2010;11(5):703–713.

65. Carr AA, Wilson R. A model of parental participation: a secondary data analysis. *School Community Journal* 1997;7(2):9–25.

66. Lopez GR, Scribner JD, Mahitivanichcha K. Redefining parental involvement: lessons from high-performing migrant-impacted schools. *American Educational Research Journal* 2001; 38(2):253–288.

67. McKay MM, Atkins MS, Hawkins T, Brown C, Lynn CJ. Inner-city African American parental involvement in children's schooling: racial socialization and social support from the parent community. *American Journal of Community Psychology* 2003;32(1-2):107–114.

68. Education Development Center. *Strategies for Engaging Refugee and Immigrant Families.* Newton, MA: Education Development Center; 2011: Available at http://sshs.promoteprevent.org/webfm_send/2254.

69. Shumow L, Harris W. Teachers' thinking about home-school relations in low-income urban communities. *School Community Journal 2000;*10(1):9–24.

For more information please contact

Centers for Disease Control and Prevention
1600 Clifton Road NE, Atlanta, GA 30333
Telephone: 1-800-CDC-INFO (232-4636)
TTY: 1-888-232-6348
E-mail: cdcinfo@cdc.gov Web: www.cdc.gov
Publication Date: Revised January 2013